Love Your Slim Self

Gena M. Rotas
Revised 2015

Love Your Slim Self

or

"How To Stop Trying And Start Succeeding"

Dedicated to:

My dear friend Beverly Klegraefe...

Who found life a dance,
laughter a blessing
and love the only "diet" that works!

Table of Contents

Chapter 1 - What's It All About

Chapter 2 - Comfort

Chapter 3 - Fat Is Only A Three-letter Word

Chapter 4 - **Love Your Slim Self**, Especially With Medical Conditions

Chapter 5 - Stop And Breathe

Chapter 6 - Breathe, You Deserve It

Chapter 7 - This Book is Different

Chapter 8 - Willing vs. Willingness

Chapter 9 - Let Go First

Chapter 10 - **Love Your Slim Self** Out Of Guilt

Chapter 11 - No Scales, Just Feel It

Chapter 12 - One Thing At A Time: You Choose

Chapter 13 - Tune Into Thin

Chapter 14 - I Talk To Me

Chapter 15 - What You See Is What You Get

Chapter 16 - Messages From Me To Me: Affirmations

Chapter 17 - Do You Talk To Yourself?

Chapter 18 - **Love Your Slim Self** in The Now

Chapter 19 - Thank Your Fat Self

Chapter 20 - Match Your Pictures

Chapter 21 - Theater Tickets To Your Mind

Chapter 22 - Seeing Is Believing

Chapter 23 - Believing Is Achieving, Activate Your **"ACTASIF"**

Chapter 24 - Whales

Chapter 25 - Hold That Line

Chapter 26 - As I Move And Breathe

Chapter 27 - Commencement Rose

Introduction

This little book has not found its way into your world by accident. No doubt the title intrigued you, causing you to think, "Now, that's a new twist on an old problem!"

The original idea for this book evolved from a program I designed many years ago called "Thin from Within" where I coached my clients into losing weight in an easy and comfortable way. At that time, relentless pressure from the media to lose weight quickly bombarded printed and broadcast materials, we read and heard about diet pills and diet drinks, liquid lunches and starvation diets. Advertisements for quick weight loss with the promise of "keeping it off," led to discouraging results that often caused people to gain back more weight than they had lost.

It became obvious that losing weight was not the problem. The real issue was whether or not a person believed he or she deserved to be successful and worthy of being slim, healthy and fit. Their inner voice and self-image needed new awareness and an overhaul.

"Thin from Within" approached weight loss differently, and my clients learned how to become both gentle and consistent while changing their thinking and beliefs. They learned strategies for reducing stress and anxiety and soon they could visualize themselves as slim, healthy and fit.

The process did not promise overnight results. It took more time than those 30-day diets and required a personal commitment to change. They listened to audiotapes, at home, twice a day, where directed to sit in a comfortable chair, and listen to a guided relaxation procedure which, helped them to re-design the pictures of themselves they had in their minds. The only personal commitment was to attend a coaching session, at least once a week, to support their subtle changes and successful progress toward personal health and reasonable weight loss.

For a reason I've since forgotten, I chose to follow a different path for a while, and the "Thin from Within" program moved to the back shelf. My passion for helping people become healthy again was inspired by my personal health struggles. After having surgery on a disk in my neck, I suffered a stroke. During my recovery, I began a serious quest for wellness. I found a nutritional supplement that worked for me and supported my journey towards feeling better. And even though my health was improving, I noticed that my inner self was having a heck of a time staying congruent with my wish for wellness. I began to pay attention to the energy needed to be patient and learn to love myself.

My efforts to incorporate "Thin from Within" with my new awareness of the importance of self-love came together and exploded in my head. The message I wanted to bring to people was the coaching I explain in **Love Your Slim Self.** Loving one self remains the cornerstone for any change.

As I continue to collect wisdom and ideas for future titles of continuing to love yourself, you can look for more books in the series. You are brighter than you think, and Love Your Smart Self will reinforce your brilliance. We are all braver than we seem, so Love Your Strong Self will showcase your inner strength. I am looking forward to expanding my personal motto, which is, "If it isn't any fun, find another way to do it" and the title of that book is Love Your Silly Self.

Welcome to my world of exploration and anticipation of the joys that life has to offer. You will have to make an effort, but you will reap many benefits and rewards. Think of participation as if you were in an amusement park for grown-ups. As you ride through this little book, you will begin to understand that YOU, and only you, hold the keys to your success. Not only will you learn who you are, but you also will begin to understand what self-love feels like. When you begin to love yourself, you will easily figure out what you want.

Inside of our amusement park, I've dropped you off in line. You've got your ticket in hand and this little book is your guide. Enjoy the journey of loving yourself because you will experience the ride of a lifetime!

I'll see you at your destination!

With love and laughter,

Gena

Chapter 1
What's It All About?

Are you laughing at the idea of even imagining a "slim self?" Are you asking yourself right now, "How could I even think of myself as slim, when I have been struggling with weight for most of my life?" If you can't imagine a slim self, then take that adjective and make it a verb, <u>SLIMMING</u> yourself and LOVING the results?

Can you begin to imagine yourself getting slimmer? Can you picture yourself in that outfit you have hidden in the back of the closet? Can you think about what you felt like when you were slimmer than you are now? Are you beginning to have a vision of yourself at a lighter weight? Do you want to give up thinking that you are FAT, OVERWEIGHT, OBESE, HEFTY, HAVE THUNDER THIGHS or any of the negative ideas you have internalized over your lifetime?

If the answer is YES, then you are on your way to creating something wonderful in your life. However it must be an unequivocal YES. No cheating on this one because what you think about does not count calories; it just is. When you realize the significance and the power of your thinking and your thoughts, you will be amazed at the many things that can change.

If NO is your answer; if you are not ready to Stop thinking about your fatness and overweight problem; if you are not willing to give up the "critical self," the "judging self," and the "hard on yourself" self, then we have to do some more creative problem-solving. It is not impossible for you to achieve a slim self; you just have to want it, desire it and <u>believe you deserve to have what you want</u>. Some of us have to be WILLING TO BE WILLING, you can add as many WILLINGS as you would like. Give yourself time to accept that someday you will arrive at YES.

Let's now take the YES and move to the LOVE piece. Here, you certainly can come to an understanding of compassion and empathy. Start by thinking of your best friends, loved ones, children, or relatives whom you cherish and who love you back.

Can you remember the feeling of loving those people, of caring for them, of saying words and doing things for them? Can you conjure up the feeling about how much you cared, no matter what happened, and how you were there for them and would always go that extra mile?

Take that feeling, the one of love, care, compassion, empathy, and kindness, and hold on to your seatbelt. I am going to ask you to do something with that feeling you just recreated. Can you sense that feeling of love and compassion in your body? Can you feel it in your heart? Can you make it stronger when you think of how much you truly love those people?

Now, take that feeling and pour it all over yourself. That's right. Simply take the feeling as if it were a glorious waterfall and allow it to bathe you in its love. Now there you have it: **Love Your Slim Self**. You're off to a great start!

DISCLAIMER: This is the first how-to book you will ever read that starts out by telling you to stop trying!

First, you need to understand this book is not about "losing weight." If you lose something you want to find it, and if you don't believe that, just think about the number of pounds you've lost and then found again.

NOW LET THAT THOUGHT GO.

Today is the last time to reflect on weight loss programs that never worked in the past. I'm telling you right now that those programs failed you. You did not fail them. They just weren't right for you. Among other things, they emphasized just what you want to avoid: that awful teeth-gritting, hand-clenching element called willpower. Willpower isn't power at all, because "willing" is all about trying too hard, and trying is pointless.

With all your past efforts, the focus has been wrong, just like a camera that is aimed to the right of your shoulder instead of on you. The focus is now on you, the entire you, and I want you to know that weight is a smaller part of you than you have ever dreamed.

After years of always trying too hard, there is a way for you to experience this slimming process that is COMFORTABLE and EASY, and most importantly in a way that is guaranteed to transform your life.

Love Your Slim Self is about a change in FEELINGS. It is not about rigid eating schedules and food lists. It is not about physical, emotional, and psychological exhaustion.

There is an unspoken myth that if you really want success; you have to fight for it. You have to give up the pleasures of life, be denied, be deprived, and struggle for success. Well, I'm here to tell you... That's Hogwash!

In this program, there is an acknowledgement that in the past you have tried too hard, much too hard! There IS an uncomplicated way to successful weight loss and a lifetime of weight control, and this is it.

Love Your Slim Self is learning how to allow you, at a super-conscious level, to create a new image, one that is absolutely necessary for positive change. Comfortable weight loss will then happen naturally.

Love Your Slim Self makes it possible for you to operate a previously hidden series of controls and to activate some that have not existed before, at least not until now.

Love Your Slim Self sends a message to your computer-like brain. Once you learn to operate it, and then trust it, there'll be no stopping you.

Love Your Slim Self is a wonderful shift of feelings.

In comparison to reading music note by note and counting every beat, **Love Your Slim Self** is like flying on the wings of a song.

Love Your Slim Self is like driving on cruise control. You still are in charge of the machine, but it's EASY and COMFORTABLE.

All that trying in your past has not been wasted. Have you ever noticed that you can gather a lot of information and not absorb the facts until suddenly, when you learn one more thing, everything comes together? **Love Your Slim Self** can do that for you with all you've learned through past experiences, and make it automatic, thus EASY, COMFORTABLE, and JOYOUS.

Love Your Slim Self is an automatic, educated instinct and gives you that built-in confidence. Trust me, you'll like learning to trust your body and your instincts.

Chapter 2
COMFORT

Comfortable goes with easy. Let's talk about comfort, the last thing you expect on a slimming program. Paradoxically, the more comfort you can create for yourself, the more smoothly the program will move along. COMFORTABLE is a new and different word for weight loss, and EASY is the most successful way to do anything.

Whenever you try too hard to do something, you become tense and rigid, but everything comes more easily when you relax. You are the only one who can identify your comfort level and you'll learn more about that in upcoming chapters.

Let's take the business of dining in a certain place. Most weight-loss and behavior modification programs (and this isn't one of them) command you to eat in one place, all the time. The authors automatically assume that if you dare to eat outside of the prescribed spot, you will lose control. Where is it written that you are forbidden to sip a long, cool drink as you bathe luxuriously? The very fact that you're pampering yourself means the desire to satisfy yourself with edibles will dwindle.

Once you learn you can trust yourself, you may choose to eat in any spot you wish. As you begin to understand that you are in control not the doctor, not your mother, not your spouse, but you, either stuffing or starving yourself will become silly behaviors.

Your appetite will arrive at the **Love Your Slim Self** level, a place where both your desire for slimness and your eating behavior will merge into success. At that same spot, you will be urged to consider yourself worth pampering, will learn how to discover what actually pleasures you, and you will discover what rewards you can achieve by giving yourself what you really want.

This is not a self-love that becomes narcissistic; all that is too obsessive and just too much work. Work is the last thing you want to do. Anybody who's ever been on a diet has "tried" to stay on it.

"Try" is a word from the past! "Try" is an old tape.

Here you are simply going to "give it a go!"

"Perhaps we shall learn, as we pass through this age, that the "other self" is more powerful than the physical self we see when we look into the mirror."

- -Napoleon Hill, Think and Grow Rich

Chapter 3
FAT IS ONLY A THREE-LETTER WORD

FAT is only a three-letter word, not an epithet. The National Association to Advance Fat Acceptance (NAAFA) has helped us all by teaching society to use the word "fat." Fat is a descriptive word--- like tall, short, or tan. It need not be fraught with emotion. NAAFA believes that freedom to use the word "fat" is a big step towards acceptance, not of fat, but of self.

One of the problems is that overweight people tend to always visualize fat. What if I told you it was just as easy for them to visualize thin? No amount of visualization will change one's eyes from blue to brown, but "fat" can change to "thin," sometimes with little more than a shift in thinking.

"I can't eat that because it will..."

What?

"....make me fat."

It will do just that unless you learn to **Love Your Slim Self**.

What do you think about every time you put a spoonful of food into your mouth? Every time you chew? Every time you smell food? Every time you think of food in any form?

Love Your Slim Self means taking those moments and turning them inside out. Visualize yourself as slim, thin, healthy, fit, energetic, whatever word most appeals to you. **Love Your Slim Self** means intensifying those moments.

Perhaps those fat-thoughts might be fleeting, but they have been around for many years. Fat-thoughts represent an established habit, and you can always challenge and change a habit. **Love Your Slim Self** means using new patterns of thinking as pleasant antidotes to that previous poison. Now, change your thoughts about food to, "Everything I eat turns to energy, health, and fitness."

"You yourself, as much as anybody in the entire universe deserve your love and affection.

--Buddha

CHAPTER 4
LOVE YOUR SLIM SELF... ESPECIALLY WITH MEDICAL CONDITIONS

Even if you have restricted food plans for medical conditions (diabetes, hypoglycemia, allergies, etc.) you can embark on a plan to **Love Your Slim Self**.

A case history:

On the day Janet embarked on what she found to be the most relaxing weight-losing program she had ever encountered, she learned she had diabetes. She was devastated, but most of all she felt a different and challenging limitation.

Just when she saw herself free of food issues, she received a list of restricted foods. This was only a temporary setback though. The day she turned the problem over to Loving Her Slim Self, her life began to turn around. Within the framework of her prescribed food program, she began to apply **Love Your Slim Self** methods. She found it easy and comfortable to choose foods from the prescribed list, if and only if, she relaxed first. What she learned is that the foods themselves, while they had to correspond to the "diet," were not the issue.

Here is Ann, who tells her story about a therapy group in which she was involved:

"We were dealing with feelings, food discussions, and behavior modification. I got to the point where I burst into violent crying when the food issue came up, finally blurting, 'It's just too hard; everything is too hard!' "

Easy and comfortable are new words to most people. After years of trying, it is only recently that easy and comfortable are becoming commonplace instead of "trying hard." Compulsive trying can trigger a failure mechanism and offset the success button. Contrary to what you have been conditioned to believe, one massive TRY can cancel a series of successes. The next time you are advised to try, substitute the words "start" or "begin" or just "give it a go," and see how they change your outlook immediately.

The reason Thomas Edison accomplished the impossible was that he relaxed as he went along. Rather than trying hard, and getting frustrated, he would slow down and even take a nap, trusting that the answers would show up. He had unwavering faith and would begin again and again and again. He made hundreds of attempts and his inventions changed the world.

CHAPTER 5
STOP AND BREATHE

Before you go any further, it is important to "BREATHE." That's right, "BREATHE!" Not just a regular breath but a deep, full, comforting breath.

The air around us is more than oxygen; it is our life force, the prana the chi, yet so many of us never take advantage of it.

It's like having $1,000 to spend on a present for your self and spending only $100. The truth is, there is plenty of air for everyone and you can always take as much as you want and need. It's one of the few things in life that's always free, so indulge!

Put the book down, and take a deep comfortable breath. Feel the new energy; freshness and vitality fill your body. Literally drink in the life force around you.

As you slowly exhale, feel yourself feeling refreshed, alive and relaxed. Now you're ready for the next thought.

You will be reminded throughout the book to…. "BREATHE!"

The more you participate, the more you breathe, the more comforting it becomes.

Comfort is a good thing, and the more the better, so enjoy!

The breath is abundant, life affirming, and FREE.

So go ahead, "BREATHE!"

Just Breathe!

CHAPTER 6
BREATHE... YOU DESERVE IT

Can DESERVING be a stumbling block for many people who struggle with change? Can you stop and take a simple, full, relaxing breath? When you do stop, and just breathe, do you hear an inner voice that says, "you aren't worthy enough to take the time away from what really needs to be done" and so you don't take a slow conscious breathe?

The more you **Love Your Slim Self**, the more you will realize you are deserving. Just because you are you! Here's a suggestion to help you rewrite the internal messages that often cause discouragement when you move toward change. Take a moment to complete the information in the statement below.

"I deserve to be my ideal weight of_____."

"I deserve to be my ideal size _____."

How does it feel when you reread it to yourself?

Is some inner parent figure saying, "You don't deserve to go to the party." "You don't deserve any dinner or dessert." "You don't deserve friends." "You don't deserve love"

If you fall into that trap you will most likely finish the statements with "Because I...," which will ultimately lead to discouragement and a closet full of guilt.

The truth is that just because you may have grown several sizes beyond your ideal size, you don't need to be punished. Punishing yourself is the worst thing to do. Rewards are much more appropriate.

You can reward yourself by realizing and accepting that you deserve to be your ideal weight and size. Then you will get your just desserts. Your just desserts may be the acceptance and love you have not been able to receive because you thought you had to be punished. Eventually, your just desserts will prove to be your ideal weight and size, and much, much more.

"To be beautiful means to be yourself. You don't need to be accepted by others. You need to accept yourself."

--Thich Nhat Hanh

CHAPTER 7
THIS BOOK IS DIFFERENT

If you are like the rest of us, by now you have read at least thirty so-called "diet books", tons of articles and columns, created calorie lists, and filed away copies of diets from friends.

This approach is not about food lists, food diaries, what you ate or didn't eat. In fact, it is vital that in order for you to achieve an ideal state of mind while eating, you enjoy and savor your food. It would be more liberating, if there were no excessive emotional baggage connected with food. Can you imagine how lovely it would be if the people at the table with you, in all shapes and sizes, would refrain from making food an issue?

Have you ever known someone who might say, "If only they wouldn't serve so much food at restaurants?"   Or someone who never misses a chance when the plate comes to remark, "Oh, my word, I could never eat that much. That's enough for a week."

It's not the fact that those statements bring attention to the "way-too-big" portion, but that it may cause a response from the other people at the table. How many would consider the same meal average? Or, perhaps be able to eat three times as much? Those statements aren't said with a conscious intention to harm, but often they make you crazy or cause you to think you would give up eating all together if you could just have your heart's desire.

Love Your Slim Self is designed to take care of situations like that. When you **Love Your Slim Self**, you don't hear distractions or hurtful comments that formerly would have loomed so large they could only make you feel conflicted by self-judgments.

When you **Love Your Slim Self**, your mind's eye is completely on your goal. At the same time, you're so relaxed that your satisfaction-meter (the feeling that says you have had enough) lights up early --and often.

Love Your Slim Self has a built-in calm and a quiet resilience that allows distressing messages to float away.

Have you ever listened to the conversation at a dinner table with complete strangers? Perhaps you attended a church supper, an awards banquet, or even a fundraising event where Instead of savoring each mouthful of the present meal, many of the diners discuss restaurants they have visited, last month's ladies auxiliary dinner, or what the menu will include for an upcoming event they are planning.

To help you remember to **Love Your Slim Self** in the midst of any situation, you might call to mind the following exercise and the feelings that accompany it. Even if you are aware of the fruitless discussions, the meal will come into perspective. You will find it easier to live in the now, which is the only road to full enjoyment.

The Exercise:

Imagine yourself in a large rowboat. You don't have to row, and the water is calm. You are carrying a large basket, and it's heavy.

The basket is loaded with things from your past; all the weight loss books, calorie sheets, diets you have ever tried, and all the anxieties you experienced while you were on them as well as the despair you felt when you went off all those diets.

The basket is a heavy load.

Now, see yourself floating on a peaceful body of water on a balmy day. As you take a deep breath and drink in the day's beauty, begin to unload your basket, one piece at a time, or just dump it upside down, whichever most appeals to you.

Take a moment, to take a breath and visualize the scene with details.

Describe the feelings that show up when you do the exercise to yourself.

There is an opportunity for you to have a feeling of relief, calm, peace and overwhelming freedom. The visualization of unloading the past can give you a new perspective for change.

Feeling freedom and calm is one of the reasons this book is different. We all look for a sense and feeling of freedom, calm and peace in our lives. These emotions can carry over during mealtimes and times that can be stressful. By learning to **Love Your Slim Self**, you can learn to summon the calmness of that day on the water where you dumped the past. In your new-relaxed state of acceptance and self-love, you can begin to make new decisions.

In the **Love Your Slim Self** mode, expect the unexpected. Instinctively you will begin to limit calories even though you are not listing or counting. Your bodily processes, undisturbed by stress, distress or turmoil, click along automatically and do their natural job.

Your Personal Notes....

Take a breath...

"*I finally stopped running away from myself. Who else is there better to be?*"

--Goldie Hawn

CHAPTER 8
WILLING vs. WILLINGNESS

Willpower is not what it's cracked up to be. Willing things to happen is a grim business, but willingness is something else.

Sometimes, if you have not learned to listen to your body, you and your body will go in opposite directions. Either that or unknowingly you are sending your body in the wrong direction. Being in ill health is a struggle whether or not you are overweight.

One of the most frequent reasons people avoid losing weight is because they are afraid they'll lose their identity. They won't be the same person. Something within them keeps saying, "I don't like change... I don't want to change... I won't change!"

Review the changes in your life. Ask yourself: Did most of them require a shift on your part? Was it a long time before you could feel comfortable with the change? The fact is, sometimes, change hurts. The changes you are about to make will feel good--all of them all the time because they come from a place of self-acceptance and love.

Moving toward these changes may feel different but in the end they will feel good. Wanting to feel good is a basic human desire.

Stop to examine your reactions to past changes. Most people find their gut reaction to change is, "I really don't want to change." Yet they still say, "I'd like to be slim. I wish I were slim." If so, it's ok, what is-is. It is important to acknowledge your thoughts because when you let those thoughts go, there is room for a new idea. Here's the best part: there's a way for your wishes to come true.

The antidote to "I don't want to change" is "I want to be WILLING to change."

Now that you have faced your real feelings honestly, you may feel some hesitation. Perhaps it is not quite as strong as the stop signal that accompanies "I don't want to change," but it may be as strong as the message you get from your car when you start up a hill. Most people own cars that work just fine unless circumstances demand that it climb a slippery hill in the dead of winter. The car doesn't stall; it just sort of coughs and whimpers along the way.

Driving your car up a slippery hill can get you talking out loud. "Come on Bessie," you might say to your auto, "You can do this," "Easy does it," "Good job," "I know we can do it," "I can see the top, we're almost there," and then when you make it, "Phew, we're at the top, thank goodness you were WILLING to give it a go!"

It's easy and comfortable to say and mean: "**I am willing to be willing to change.**" You may add as many "willings" as you need, just as you would pad a painful callous with as many layers of soft gauze as you need. It's better to add willing's than weight!

One way to declare your willingness, no matter how faint it seems at the moment, is to put your imagination to work. Some of you have been brainwashed into thinking you have no imagination, don't you believe it. If you can conjure up the joys of Christmas, the smells in the house on Thanksgiving Day or the aroma of freshly brewed coffee, you have an imagination, and you have it in 3-D!

The fact that you experience craving a certain food means your imagination is working overtime. **Love Your Slim Self** helps your imagination work FOR YOU instead of against you.

For example, when you are on a strict diet and have deprived yourself all day long, you begin to think about the doughnut you hid in the freezer, just in case you "need" it. The more you think about that doughnut and the more you tell yourself one doughnut won't hurt, the shakier your willpower becomes. Eventually, you will have a doughnut if not that afternoon then perhaps that night, after you were so "good" all day.

There are all kinds of fallacies in your thinking, but for now, just consider this: when willpower and imagination are in conflict, it is always imagination that will win. **Love Your Slim Self** can change your imagination into a tool that will create slimness instead of hunger and craving. If you are willing.

Again, this is a lot like the cruise control in your car. The cruise control won't operate without a willing driver to activate it and until you are comfortable using it, you may not appreciate its value. There are reasons you may not use it; you may think traffic is not sparse enough, you may think you'll lose control of your car, you may forget about it because you haven't used it very often and you aren't familiar with its operation, etc .

Just like your cruise control, **Love Your Slim Self** needs to be used, and the more you use it, the more automatic it will become. Imagination is just one aspect of **Love Your Slim Self**. Instead of picturing that doughnut with its texture, shape and flavor, with **Love Your Slim Self** you immediately picture the slim self you are and the entire series of wonderful scenes that go with being the **SLIM YOU**. Since the mind can focus on only one picture at a time, the slim picture takes over and banishes the other unwanted image.

Notes:

"*Love yourself enough to take the actions required for your happiness....Love yourself enough to cut yourself loose from the ties of the drama-filled past....Love yourself enough to move on!*"

--Steve Maraboli Unapologetically You

CHAPTER 9
LET GO

No matter how much you talk or think about wanting to lose those extra pounds, there is usually some hidden reason you have been holding on to the weight.

It's a little like not wanting to give up your coat when you arrive at a party. It's a nuisance to carry around but nevertheless, you keep it wrapped tightly around you and you're not exactly sure why.

That's why it's so important to **Love Your Slim Self**. When you begin to relax and enjoy the party, suddenly you will not need your coat! When you're really having fun, you may toss it on a chair because it's no longer important. What is important is having fun at the party.

The following story might make this concept clearer. Once there was a father, Alan, who was tormented by the grief over the loss of his two children who had died in a car accident five years ago. For five years he carried a heavy heart and a dark sadness. He did not want to live fully because his grief, painful as it was, represented part of his children. By holding onto the grief he was able to stop himself from feeling love, compassion and calm again. He had no intention of giving it up, or letting it go, even though he had tried many times to heal his heart.

Not for a single moment did Alan believe he deserved to ever feel free and happy again.

If you're thinking his pain is not comparable to how you feel being overweight, you're right. But the technique you use to hold onto that pain is exactly the same.

People who are overweight believe they never deserve to be their ideal weight.

"Why are you trying so hard to fit in when you were born to stand out?"

--Ian Wallace

Just breathe...

CHAPTER 10
LOVE YOUR SLIM SELF
OUT OF GUILT

"Giving myself permission to..." and "Not expecting myself to...." are words that are not a natural part of an overweight person's vocabulary. Even if you have resolved again and again to be good to yourself, you never felt you could consider your health and comfort before others.

Tell yourself, "**It is easy and comfortable for me to take care of this body**." You can **Love Your Slim Self**.

A woman named Alice decided to give herself a holiday present a more relaxed self. (Can you see how **Love Your Slim Self** was beginning to make a difference for her?) One way was to give herself permission to avoid food events for a while. Since she knew herself well enough to know that fellowship was important to her, therefore, she did not stay away from the entire meeting; she just wanted to avoid the dinner. In the past, she would succumb to the pressure and criticism of others and would have had much too much to eat.

Sometimes, when you are offered a meal, the host will feel rejected because you didn't accept the nutritious offer. Such people have a problem of their own, and you don't need to be involved in it. Avoid them temporarily, if you must. Better still, be secure in the knowledge that you can respond with tactful comments to their invitations that will warm them instead of hurt them.

Gratitude and appreciation are feelings that help make any situation calmer and more genuine. You can tell your host that their food offering must have taken special effort and that you truly appreciate the time and energy it took to make you feel so welcome. You want them to understand that there is nothing personal intended when you have to decline the offer, because your present health plan is asking you to pass for now...not forever, just for now!

One way to achieve that security is to use the tools you are learning in this program. Recognize that stress is involved, and your cue is to **SMILE ON STRESS**; then **BREATHE** and **DO** what supports your success. You'll learn more about this in the next chapter.

If you invite people to your home, you can feel comfortable announcing that only coffee and tea will be available and that it is about being together that counts. It is perfectly fine to serve as a host or hostess in ways other than preparing and serving food and there's no reason to feel guilty.

There's another tyranny that can cause guilt though. When friends meet, it doesn't need to mean eat! Where is it written that you have to do anything you don't want to do when it comes to designing your success?

Too often, friends avoid one another rather than face the pressure of temptation and guilt. When you **Love Your Slim Self**, you sail through such situations, knowing you can eat or not, and that there is no built-in rule.

Love Your Slim Self also frees you from past programming. The more you practice **Loving Your Slim Self**, the easier it is to do.

Take meal skipping; what dire predictions do you hear from your inner voices about that? What does it mean to skip breakfast or to go without having something to eat all day? You get the idea. Voices from the past attach guilt and **Love Your Slim Self** releases you from the past.

There is a difference between being guilty and feeling guilty, but both are painful and damaging. As if you're not susceptible enough to guilt, there are people in your surroundings who are experts at injecting you with guilt, especially when you're off guard.

One of the best resolutions you can make is to not feel guilty, no matter what. I know "guilt" is supposed to be a noun, but when you turn it into a verb, you can help yourself prevent many guilt trips.

It is **EASY** and **COMFORTABLE** to recognize "guilting," and to turn it off instantly.

Instead, **Love Your Slim Self**.

Notes:

"Loving yourself....does not mean being self-absorbed or narcissistic, or disregarding others. Rather it means welcoming yourself s the most honored guest in your own heart, a guest worthy of respect, a lovable companion."

--Margo Anand

CHAPTER 11
NO SCALES, JUST FEEL IT

For too long, the scale has tyrannized you.

In your new comfortable, easy program, part of **Love Your Slim Self** means that you don't have to step on a scale to get weighed.

If you follow the program, one of three things will happen; you will see you have lost weight, you might gain weight, or you may stay the same. If you are still letting the scale run your life, you will act in whatever way you have conditioned yourself to act in the past.

Overeaters Anonymous (O.A.), the group based on the principles of Alcoholics Anonymous (A.A.) and the 12-STEP Program, may have led many people from scale-control to weight-control. Overcoming scale tyranny is another way to get your eye off the problem and onto the goal. This perspective will support your efforts to take "baby-steps" and will validate your progress.

There may come a day when you will love stepping on the scale, but for now, remove that tension from your life. For one, few scales are completely accurate, and most thin people gauge their weight by how their clothes fit.

If you've ever brooded about what the scale says, there are many more constructive things to do and more reasons to do them. Once you have relaxed and taken yourself to the easy, comfortable **Love Your Slim Self** mindset, you can start to think of how easy everything is becoming. Use your imagination and picture the following activities and the positive emotion that goes with it.

Think of how wonderful it feels to:

Zip up your size (fill in your perfect size) dress.

Lean down to tie your shoes.

Stand up to zip your designer jeans, easily.

Cross your arms comfortably.

Walk away from the dinner table without feeling stuffed.

Rejoice that you can feel a bit hungry now and then.

Add your own here! _____

How about that excitement you feel in the dressing room when you try on new clothes? How do you feel wearing shorts to play tennis, or even playing tennis? Gardening? Bending? Being able to comfortably unlock the security bar on your steering wheel?

Isn't it wonderful to know you don't have to wait for some distant date to feel terrific? In **Love Your Slim Self**, you can feel terrific **NOW**, and the best thing about it is that the more you practice these scenes in your mind's eye, the nearer the reality becomes. All because it's not magic, it's you! The mind begins to create what you visualize and the more you create these pictures, the easier it becomes.

If your car is serviced frequently, it is more apt to run smoother than the car the mechanic never sees. When your kitchen floor is dirty, you have to scrub, scour, scrape, and shine it until you feel it's clean again. But, if the floor is cared for regularly, isn't it easy to keep it looking the way you like it just by giving it frequent once-overs?

If your relaxation and visualization processes are kept in frequent operation, they soon become automatic responses. Using the technique of visualization, you can guide your way to slimness all day and all night. It's easy, and it's comfortable.

S.O.S. or **Smile on Stress** is an easy strategy. In your mind, see yourself smiling. The tiny muscles on your face will respond without you knowing. Something happens in your brain that sends a signal to release the hormones that help you relax. Then, take a deep easy breath and say to yourself, **"My thoughts are clear and my body is relaxed."** As you exhale, imagine warm energy flowing throughout your body. When you smile on the inside, the outside world changes. The same smile works when you encounter a stressful situation. The stress triggers the inner smile, and the inner smile triggers the freedom from stress. The conscious mind will remind you that you can do only one thing at a time: stress or smile.

If you experiment with only this strategy, you will have a preview of the success you can expect with **Love Your Slim Self**. When you smile in response to stress, you are **Loving Your Slim Self**.

Breathe.......

"Find the love you seek, by first finding the love within yourself. Learn to rest in that place within you that is your true home."-- Sri Ravi Sahnkar

---

40

CHAPTER 12

ONE THING AT A TIME. YOU CHOOSE

The mind can only focus on one picture at a time. You have a choice whether to think negative or positive thoughts and both thoughts take the same energy. Both thoughts can bring changes in our bodies and bodily functions.

When we are thinking about food, language plays a major role in our thinking. The negative phrases and associations made around eating and food often set us up for frustration and failure.

Here are some of the more common phrases: "Pigging out" "Wolfing down" "Chewing like a cow" "The clean plate club" "Super-sizing your drink" "I'm so full, I feel like I will burst" "I could eat a horse," and "If I don't get something to eat soon, I will die of starvation" "Who cares anyway, I might as well eat all night."...

Do you hear the negative energy and see the discouraging imagery?

Your mind works in pictures and each one of the negative statements sets a picture of discouragement in the personal vision of yourself.

Negativity is one of your worst enemies, and here's why; when you are told to stop doing something what happens most frequently is that you cannot stop. This is because the mind is just unable to reverse the negative message. You remember and do what you heard last. When you tell the kids to "stop fighting," they go on fighting for a longer time. Shout to the kids on the way to school,

---

"Don't forget your homework," and the last words they hear are "forget your homework." The mind does not have the skill to turn the statement into the positive before it is too late, and so you have to make an extra trip to school to bring the homework they forgot.

Orders are uncomfortable for anyone. No one likes to be told what to do, and it is almost as if people want to get even with the authority by not doing what the authority figure says. How many times have you reminded people to do something and they still forget? Are you aware of your language?

"Don't spill the drink," "Don't forget to make your bed," "Don't yell at me," "Don't forget the milk."

The absent-minded person tends to hear only "**forget the milk**," so he comes home empty-handed. Not on purpose, it's just that the mind can only entertain one thought at a time. Either forget, or don't, and usually it is the last statement the mind hears.

When you see the red stoplight, you automatically step on the brake pedal and your mind confirms, "**STOP**." It doesn't say, "Do not keep going!" At that instant, when you see the STOP sign, you are not thinking of the grocery list or what you will wear to the party tomorrow night. Your mind can only think and focus on one thought at a time. For a red light, it is to bring the car to a stop.

Since the mind can focus on only one thing at a time, it is best to keep the command positive. A negative command will only get a negative response. If you tell the kids, "Be careful and don't drop the dishes," chances are much stronger you will be cleaning the floor before those plates reach the counter.

Try, "don't slam the door; the baby's asleep," and it will take you twenty more minutes to get the baby back to sleep. When you say to yourself, "I just bought that blouse. I hope I don't get gravy on it tonight," the cleaners will appreciate your cooperation. A positive goal or positive thought will get the kind of results you deserve and desire. "Carry the dish carefully," "Close the door softly," and "Enjoy wearing that blouse" are all positive thoughts.

The same is true of trying to lose weight by dieting. When you think of dieting, you think about not being able to eat what you want, wishing for the diet to be over, longing for favorite foods, or being deprived of what you enjoy in life (food). You think of food much more often than if you weren't on a diet. When you think of the positive and begin to frame statements for your success, you begin to see the ease with which you can command your actions.

Here are some positive thoughts:

Turn off the alarm clock.

Grab that whistling kettle.

Close the window so that the floor stays dry.

Pay the man at the tollbooth.

Remove my scratchy contact lens.

Most likely, you have 50 million thoughts a day. Why spend your energy making them negative when positive thinking can lead you to success? Positive thinking can't hurt you! Just look at what negative thinking has already done to all of us:

Here are some negative one-liners:

It's going to rain and ruin our picnic.

I'm so tired I can't see straight.

I'll never get that job.

Everyone is in such a bad mood at the office.

Nothing ever gets done around here.

I never get respect.

You never appreciate anything I do.

You'll be sure to catch cold without your coat.

How stupid I am, just look at the mess.

Words create images in your mind and images trigger emotions. Emotion moves you towards actions, and actions create images, which trigger emotions, which move you towards action, etc.

Maybe you have tried to motivate yourself to lose weight by looking in the mirror and saying, "Enough already! When are you going to get down to business?"

It probably never occurred to you how much easier and pleasurable it would be to look in the same mirror, smile at the face in there and say, "You're fantastic. You're slimming down."

The results could surprise you. Certainly yelling at yourself didn't work. If you've been saying, "Everything I eat turns to fat," change the words and say, "Everything I eat turns to energy, health, and fitness."

Both sayings take the same amount of energy.

The more often you repeat the words to yourself, the truer the statement becomes. "Everything I eat turns to energy, health, and fitness." There's something about a positive approach that makes subtle changes in your mind and in your relationship to food. Often, it results in the consumption of fewer calories. There are studies to suggest that accompanying physiological changes take place when the mind set is altered. Too many people adopt "Don't eats" as their weight-losing program. **Love Your Slim Self** offers a list of "Do's." Most of them are far removed from food, and thus help you achieve successful results.

You can only choose one thing at a time. When you say "No" to the negative thinking, critical self-talk, harsh judgments, you say "Yes" to your lovely slim self.

Notes:

"*When you truly love yourself, you are enough. Your happiness and well-being become a top priority.*"

--Annette Vaillancourt

CHAPTER 13
TUNE INTO THIN

For so long you have been conditioned to carry your body around without trusting it. And now you know that the body doesn't lie. In fact, the body tells it all.

Today, we live in a time when we work too hard, play too hard, and forget to take care of ourselves. The only time we ever listen to our body is when we have an accident or become too ill to function. Even then, we tend to think it's a germ that's to blame when, in reality, it's the body's way of bringing the rushing train to a stop before it goes over the cliff of health and wellbeing.

Two alarms sound in your body. The first is to help you notice that you are getting too tired and you'd better slow down. If you listen to the first, you can usually forestall the second. How many times have loved ones told you to slow down? The second is that you are already exhausted, and if you don't stop instantly, there will be trouble ahead. Trouble comes in many forms: an accident, a disease, a hospitalization, a headache, a long-lasting cold, or even a skin breakout.

Talking to your body is just as powerful as listening to what your body tells you. Not only do you have to learn to listen to your body, but also you have to be vigilant about what you say to yourself.

"If I eat that doughnut, it will go directly to my hips!" Sound familiar?

The mind-body language we use can become a significant strategy for re-educating and liberating the people on perpetual diets.

Love Your Slim Self uses the body talk of becoming slim from the inside out. Tuning into your inner voice and listening to what makes your heart sing will help you find **FULFILLERS.**

Sarah's fulfiller might be a cream puff, and Mike's might be a cucumber. You won't know until you listen to your body. Sometimes, when the message is unclear, you might want to postpone eating until you really hear it. It's easy to do this if you listen.

You can experiment with being still enough to register a feeling and then notice the thoughts you are having before you make a decision to eat something. Say to yourself: "Is there a feeling that I can identify?" Such as: sad, mad, glad, afraid, or even happy? "Can I wait just a few minutes before I unconsciously begin eating again?" Maybe post those questions on sticky notes around your world and remind yourself they are your own personal coaching clues.

The idea isn't to eat everything in sight. It's just that you may never have learned that it's okay to experience sensuous pleasure from the food you eat. In fact, once you allow yourself to believe you deserve that pleasure you will be free from the pressures surrounding food.

The average dieter is in prison following rules made by somebody else. The average dieter thinks that if he or she does not abide by every rule, if he chooses to take a bite of something wrong, he's **BAD**. If he chooses the "right" food, he's **GOOD**. This cycle only leads to stumbling feelings of helplessness and discouragement. There's nothing more devastating than believing we've been BAD.

THIS IS WHY THE SYSTEM FAILED YOU.

All those systems of dieting fostered juvenile value systems, good and bad foods, good and bad eating, good and bad cravings, and sent them far into your adult years. Right now, test yourself. Make a list of your favorite foods and any others you can think of in ten seconds. Then classify them all as either bad or good.

Do you really want to perpetuate the Good/Bad cycle? If not, ask yourself if looking at things as either "good" or "bad" is a realistic value system for you. If you're on the **Love Your Slim Self** wavelength, you'll laugh at yourself and shatter a myth you have believed in for years. There is no "good" or "bad," there just is!

Look in the mirror. Take a deep breath and say, "I'm terrific!"

This suggestion is a powerful way to dispel the misconception that you are BAD in any way, shape, or form! There is preciousness in you that is aching to be acknowledged, and it must start with you. Take this idea seriously. You are terrific just because you are!

At first looking in the mirror and saying positive words to your self may seem silly, but gradually such behavior will become automatic. Being positive in your words to yourself will become a way to **Love Your Slim Self** quickly. You are pressing the **Love Your Slim Self** button in your mind.

In this program, you are instructed to breathe. **Do it.** Once you have practiced the breathing exercises, you will find a single breath will move you quickly to the level where the instructions you give yourself will take root at a surprising rate of speed. Progress will materialize just like the automatic shifting of a car's engine. Instead of wondering about it, your body will take over and respond to the new ways of thinking, just like blinking. You don't think about the need for moisture in your eyes, your body does that automatically for you and it brings comfort. If you practice breathing, then think of yourself as "fabulous," eventually the thought and the calmness will bring comfort to you.

Once you agree to tune in to your wishes and your appetite, you will find yourself asking questions such as these:

Am I really hungry, or am I thirsty, or tired?

Would a little nap do as well as a snack?

Is what I really want that delicious feeling of snuggling into bed with my softest pillow and drifting off?"

"Delicious" is a word that applies to many other things besides food. It applies to warm, comforting feelings you can always use more of that.

When the practice of talking to your body is still new, a wonderful way to get in touch with it is to write out the dialogue. You might even want to give your body a name, so the dialogue will feel natural. You can be Young Self, "**YS**" or Grown-up Self, "**GUS**." The names will yield some wonderful and surprising results.

When you learn to listen to and laugh along with the body that the dialogue becomes instructive.

Remember, it is **EASY** and **COMFORTABLE** to let the dialogue take shape. Step out of your own way and let the thoughts flow naturally. You will be surprised and even delighted to hear what your body has to say. If you have the least bit of hesitation, try starting it like a letter:

DEAR BODY,

... Allow Body to answer, as he/she will.

CHAPTER 14

I TALK TO ME

Here is an example of a dialogue between a young self "YS" and a Grown-up Self "GUS". Some comments were very short and filled an immediate need; others were longer. See if you identify with any of the script.

Young Self: "YS" / Grown Up Self: "GUS"

GUS: I really want to have a talk with you.

YS: I know. You want to say you're sick of this whole (dieting) business.

GUS: That's right.

YS: I told you we would work together.

GUS: But I get so discouraged. I think it's entirely your fault.

YS: What's my fault?

GUS: You and your faulty chemistry!

YS: Even if that's possible or believable, it still takes two of us. I can't operate without you! You had bad habits, and you needed to change them. It doesn't matter that other people seem to be abusing their bodies. So what if what they do makes your habits look as if you're wearing a halo! That thinking doesn't melt away any weight.

GUS: I'm sure you're right, but...

YS: But nothing! Just because you've called me "YS" doesn't mean I'm entirely stupid. I knew what to do and what was right for me long before you became GUS. You did, too, but it was programmed out of you.

GUS: Are you trying to punish me?

YS: That would punish both of us.

GUS: Then what shall we do?

YS: Trust me. I'll help you, but every time you get discouraged, I hurt. How would you like it if I fell apart every time you needed to depend on me? That's how it is for me when you fall apart and get discouraged. We need to work together. If I commit myself to you, I expect the same commitment and consistency in return.

GUS: O.K. And thanks.

YS AND GUS: On to victory!

In another conversation, GUS didn't know what to talk about, but YS said it was patience.

GUS: I thought I was very patient!

YS: I know. You thought you were doing right with "if at first you don't succeed, try, try again." That had been drummed into you, and when some things never worked out, you got so discouraged.

GUS: Now I think there are different ways of trying. The kind of trying I was into was control, which only works for a while. Then I began trying by relaxing. It's no wonder people say "Lighten up," when they see someone tense and over-trying.

YS: You got it! As they say.

GUS: But about patience, even if I could be patient, the doctors and society don't want to wait and that makes me upset not to be achieving, and I get panicky.

YS: Right. When will you learn? If you get upset about those things, it becomes harder to relax. If you don't relax, there's no harmony. If there's no harmony, there's no being thin. Come on!

GUS: Don't you think it's funny that you're doing most of the advising?

YS: Not at all. We both know the truth, but you keep forgetting it, or submerging it. It's like that song, "The more we get together, together, together, the more we get together, the happier we'll be."

GUS: Have you noticed that the last two times we talked, I had a hard time beginning?

YS: It's important that you give yourself permission to speak and that you opened the conversation even without knowing what you wanted to talk about.

GUS: I suppose, but who is the authority figure here, you or me?

YS: Don't you know?

GUS: I guess it has to be both of us to work (long sigh).

YS and GUS: On towards the goal.

Read through the conversations again, and give yourself a chance to marvel at the spontaneity and the course they took. They followed a pattern: doubt, uncertainty, then assurance, humor, some conflict, and a coming together at the end, as both selves recognize their common goal.

Perhaps you might try the same strategy and have that heartfelt conversation with your inner self, who is just aching to be heard. It will teach you something and you might be delighted by the surprise. Remember, the Body knows everything, and it never forgets!

Just Breathe......

"*Our entire life...consists ultimately in accepting ourselves as we are>*"

--Jean Anouih

CHAPTER 15
WHAT YOU SEE IS WHAT YOU GET

What you can see in your mind's eye, you can achieve. See your success and it's yours.

Try this exercise:

Imagine you want a lemon. Now imagine yourself going into the kitchen, opening the refrigerator, pulling open the door and reaching for a nice, yellow, juicy lemon. See yourself picking up a knife and slicing into the lemon. You can almost feel the spray of vapor. The smell is fragrant and clean. You can almost taste it at this point.

Now take a slice of the lemon, and bite into it. More taste. Lick the lemon, and feel your glands tighten. If you have been using your imagination, you can actually feel as if you have eaten a lemon. Some people say they begin to feel the saliva in their mouth react to the tartness of the fruit. The mouth waters as if the person was actually sucking a lemon.

Long, ago, when medicine was still young, patients who suspected they had the mumps were told to suck on a lemon. If their glands were painful, they knew for sure it was the mumps. You can achieve that same strong feeling of tartness and sour pull on your glands just by using your imagination.

Your mind works in pictures, and your subconscious cannot tell the difference between what is real and what is clearly imagined.

That is why you can almost taste the lemon.

The lemon illustration makes it easier to demonstrate how the two sides of your brain work. The left side of your brain thinks in words and logical sequences, uses numbers, and is very structured. The right side uses images, pictures, feelings, and impressions. It is where the artist and the daydreamer in each of us live.

Remember when you were young and in school sitting in a boring class and staring out the window. The teacher told you to, "Stop daydreaming." That was really the left side of the teacher's brain scolding the right side of yours.

Daydreaming is what reality is made of.

Love Your Slim Self is the cruise control to the right side of the brain. By asking you to visualize and imagine yourself the way you would like to be, you are setting up the mechanism for your success. When you begin to sense your success and feel your confidence, you begin to believe in your ability to have anything you desire.

As you practice using your natural ability to visualize and imagine success, you are preparing your mind for the moment when everything seems to fall into place. Some call it the "Ah-ha response." Others simply say, "It finally clicked."

Right-brain thinking often requires more patience than the left. Remember, right-brain thinking is in images and it takes a while for the brain to put your thought into words. If you should become impatient with your progress, think of this:

Imagine you are preparing a dinner for your family. You have four pots on the stove, and something in the oven. Although you have planned to have all your cooking done at the same time, it is inevitable that some foods may finish cooking before the others. Some dishes need more time to sit and simmer.

You are willing to wait for the complete meal because that is the picture you have of serving the full dinner.

When you are impatient with your weight loss, you know that it is simmering on the back burner of your right brain. You need to remain confident that your journey will finish.

Now BREATHE...

"It's not your job to like me....it's MINE!"

--Byron Katie

CHAPTER 16
MESSAGES FROM ME TO ME: AFFIRMATIONS

An affirmation is a statement from your conscious to your subconscious mind, which declares that a desired state of being has already come to pass. If your inner computer doesn't recognize the word "affirmations," and some do not, why not consider them just messages from me to me? These messages from me to me can accomplish what we never dreamed possible. If you doubt it, just try a few on for size and see what happens. It won't happen overnight, but the speed that change takes place will surprise you. You also can use this process for creating a more comfortable experience when fear and anxiety are present. Remember to breathe and then believe your ability to create something different is possible. Be clear with the results you would like to manifest.

For instance, you want to be calm and relaxed going into the dentist's office. Practice the feeling of calm and relaxed before you even get there. In your imagination, you actually see yourself acting relaxed and calm. Aren't you a little surprised you can picture the change? When you make this message personal, it will impact your life. Remember the lemon exercise?

The following testimony, from Karen, shows what happened when she made the decision to apply the process when she visited her doctor:

> I really didn't believe it would work, and as the appointment grew near, I found myself more apprehensive than ever. I continued to give myself the message, gently, without urgency, even on the examining table. Then I became strangely calm.
>
> The doctor asked if I had any questions or problems. I found I really didn't. He asked me what was really on my mind, and I answered, 'Nothing.' Then I began to laugh.
>
> Finally, he said, 'Well, I think you do have something on your mind; but anyway, there's something different about you today. I just can't put my finger on it.' I, of course, knew exactly what it was. The affirmation, or message from me to me was in operation, and I didn't have to do anything. In fact, the less I did, the more operational the message became.

Choose your message. "It is **EASY** and **COMFORTABLE** for me to _____ (now just fill in the blank)."

CHAPTER 17
DO YOU TALK TO YOURSELF?

Do you know it's healthy to talk to yourself?

Talking to yourself is normal and can be healthy when you choose to talk in a positive voice. It all depends on what you say and how you say it. Remember that you are in charge of the self-talk and you choose either positive or negative thoughts, which orchestrate the inner dialogue.

Do you really want to reinforce the message that you're stupid? You do so every time you drop or forget something, and you berate yourself by saying: "How stupid!"

Perhaps you haven't listened to yourself lately. Below are some examples of negative self-talk. If you identify with any of them, then you are in the right place to begin to find ways to change these negative remarks into positive remarks.

SITUATIONAL REMARKS

You spilled gravy on your tie. **What a slob! I knew I'd do that!**

You turned down the wrong street. **Wouldn't you know it?**

You locked the key in the car. **How dumb can I be?**

You failed to keep a date. **Forgetful me! Absent minded!**

You drop a dish, or you trip. **Clumsy!**

You must admit that sometimes, just sometimes, you might do something that you think is "stupid". You might spill the milk, drop the glass, trip on the rug, eat seven doughnuts, or get spaghetti sauce on your shirt, "How stupid of me!"

The words you say to yourself elicit an emotional response, which is almost out of your control. You may experience a feeling of embarrassment or shame. It may be a warm but disturbing energy that rises in your belly, explodes around your heart, and shoots directly to your brain. And you then feel lousy.

Let's consider deleting the word "stupid" from your consciousness. Replace it with an acronym that just might give you permission to love yourself unconditionally.

S.T.U.P.I.D. means:

"Some Trip Ups Postpone Intelligent Decisions"

Write it on a card and post it all around your world. Memorize it, so the next time you use the word "stupid", it is not a direct insult to yourself.

You can feel better about **Not Being Perfect**. Isn't that a relief? In fact, it is best to avoid perfection altogether. Just keep going. Pick yourself up, have a little chuckle, pat yourself on the back, and say, "Oops, that was a trip up".

The truth is you talk to yourself in ways that would make you furious if you observed anyone else speaking to you in that manner. It's as if you are holding two telephone receivers to your ears and listening to an opposite message in each ear. The chatter can become destructive and you begin to feel defeated. Be easy on yourself. Listen to what you are actually saying and if you are ready for change, your new encouraging words will usher that negative self-talk away.

Listen closely, so you can simply **Love Your Slim Self**.

CHAPTER 18
LOVE YOUR SLIM SELF ...
IN THE NOW

Love Your Slim Self means thinking in a different way, and thinking in the "here and now." You have probably heard about **Mindfulness**, which is, living in the present moment, on purpose, in a particular way and without judgment.

Orienting yourself around this new attitude of **Love Your Slim Self** will allow you to forgive the past and look forward to the future. That's a relief! Just think how delicious (this time it is a deliberate reference to food) it would be to be able to "let go of" the guilt, shame, regret, pain, and sorrow of what happened earlier.

At this point you might be thinking: "But, I am not Slim NOW! How will just thinking differently work for me?"

Just asking this question is a very important beginning to the change that will take place on the inside of who you are in relationship to your body. It is vital that you think about loving yourself now, no matter what shape your body is in. Having the courage to actually admit that there is unconditional love for yourself will help you move past the memories and struggles you have endured. When you are thinking in the "here and now", and loving who you are, you will create a new experience each and every day. The past is over. Those negative thoughts can never hurt you again. The future is only a possibility, so your power is in the present moment.

Occasionally, however, you may hear an inner voice, an inner critic that doubts and judges the success of your intentions.

Lisa was having difficulty visualizing herself slim in the "here and now." She had a photograph of herself when she was younger. In the photo, she was in a wheelchair and was very ill. She was slim at that time in her life, but, now, the thought of being slim meant she would be ill again.

Her inner picture was equated to being ill. If slim meant to be in a wheelchair, why get slim?

She mentioned this to her husband, who quickly drew from his wallet two snapshots of a young mother, slim and attractive, after she had recovered from her illness. "Aha," she thought, "these pictures will inspire me." So she posted them on her refrigerator, thinking she had found the solution. For further inspiration, she also began looking at her wedding pictures.

Does this scenario sound familiar?

Here comes the twist. The past is over, and the photos were taken in the past; so they hold no power in the present.

Lisa's new slim self needs to emerge from a loving place inside her to the present moment.

The "here and now" means believing that you are able to **Love Your Slim Self**, the self that is already here.

When Lisa realized her challenge, she took a piece of paper and created an illustration that represented her as she was now. She put all of the wonderful encouraging words and phrases she could think of around the picture of herself.

"This is me, loving my slim self," was the caption and she added words and phrases that supported her loving herself,

unconditionally.

Healthy

Strong

Slim

Fabulous

Terrific

(and yes)

Sexy

What old photos are you keeping in front of you?

Love Your Slim Self into the here and now and the new.

Just Breathe...

"If you aren't good at loving yourself, you will have a difficult time loving anyone, since you'll resent the time and energy you give another person that you aren't even giving to yourself."

--Barbara DeAngelis

CHAPTER 19
THANK YOUR FAT SELF

Love Your Slim Self happens first on the inside so you are **PREPARED** to be slim. The first step in **Loving Your Slim Self** is to **Love Your Fat Self.** Unconditionally! Don't think you're inviting your Fat Self to stay around; rather, acknowledge who you are in this present moment.

Sometimes you might see a drawing of a slim self stepping out of the fat self, and perhaps it should be the fat self leaving the slim self.

Let's reconsider the point of origin. Some of you may have experienced grieving when your excess weight is gone. That's right, grief and mourning because you have lost something dear to you. Sometimes, the weight loss is equivalent to a whole person.

If you are not already slim from within, when you lose a hundred pounds or more, you have lost more than just weight. It could be a traumatic adjustment.

Loving Your Slim Self is to say: **"I accept myself completely as I am, here and now."**

Think of your dearest, closest friend. Have you now accepted him or her as he/she is? Eventually, we learn not to try to change a friend; that's one reason the friendship has grown.

Fat Self has been your best friend. You have needed Fat Self, or you would have bid him/her goodbye long ago. Many books go into all the reasons you clung to Fat Self. You know the reasons too, but most of you have found it too painful to pinpoint them or let them rise to your conscious mind. It hurts terribly to say you are afraid you'll disappear, sicken and die, or become like Aunt Whoever.

Some of you are sure that if you get rid of your most important possessions or you'll die.

With **Love Your Slim Self**, you keep the parts of Fat Self you still need or want. Yes, there are some desirable parts: sensuousness, softness, voluptuousness, style, rhythm, voice, delight, sense of bounteousness, sense of humor, and certainly compassion for others who are struggling because you know how it hurts to be (and feel) fat.

So, instead of bullying Fat Self, (after all, what way is that to treat a friend?), you will experience a kind parting. **Imagine this dialogue between Fat Self and Slim Self:**

SLIM SELF: Fat Self, I really want to thank you.

FAT SELF: That's a switch.

SLIM SELF: Yes, it is. I have finally realized how loyal you have been. You have comforted me, enveloped me, and warmed me when the chips were down. You have kept people from getting too close to me when I was hurting the most. You have been a moat around my castle.

FAT SELF: I only took directions from you.

SLIM SELF: That's what I'm beginning to realize. I'm the one who ordered you to get fatter, and you just obeyed. I remember when I wanted to use you as an excuse for the way some people were treating me. It's true, they did treat me badly, but I could fall back on you.

FAT SELF: I remember. That's when you said it was just because you were fat. If you were thin it would be different.

SLIM SELF: I tried to get rid of you so many times, but you kept coming back.

FAT SELF: You called me! As soon as you started out into the world alone, you felt naked and retreated, so you ran back inside.

SLIM SELF: How foolish. Most of the things I was trying to hide were already apparent to people who knew me. I thought I was traveling undercover. I was, in a way, but now it's safe to come out. I guess some of us might be called "closet thins" but we masquerade as "fat."

FAT SELF: Boy, it's good to see you a little kinder to yourself and to me!

SLIM SELF: Speaking of being kind, there's one thing that's bothering me a lot.

FAT SELF: What's that?

SLIM SELF: Well, considering the times I tried to kill you off, (ugh, I shudder when I think of it), and in the process wounded myself almost fatally, I don't know the etiquette of getting rid uh...of...uh...inviting you to leave. Is there a Fat Self heaven or what? The truth is, I'm not in the mood for grieving. Can you help me?

FAT SELF: I think so. It's a little like lending your housekeeper. Okay, so you don't have one, but if you did?

SLIM SELF: If I did, the only time I wouldn't need her would be if I went on a round-the-world cruise or some exciting thing like that. Then I'd want you back, and I really don't, want you back, that is.

FAT SELF: But you're going to be on a cruise the rest of your life, a **Love Your Slim Self** cruise, one on which thinking slim and eating slim are going to be so much a part of you, that it's doubtful you would ever need me again. There'll be no room for me in your life anymore.

SLIM SELF: That's true. I think I'll miss you but not enough to summon you back. In that case...Go!

FAT SELF: You don't pull any punches, do you? It will take me a little while to get my things together, so I'll have to move out gradually. Is that O.K.?

SLIM SELF: Just so you go!

FAT SELF: Don't worry about it! No problem! Fortunately, my services are very much in demand. There's no unemployment in my field. In fact, that guy around the corner whose wife just left him is an excellent candidate, or that little kid down the street whose parents keep stuffing him with doughnuts whether he's hungry or not. Better they should use kisses, and not the candy kind!

SLIM SELF: Thanks again for all your help and comfort.

FAT SELF: It sure is nice to be appreciated.

Smiling, they both wave good-bye.

CHAPTER 20

MATCH YOUR PICTURES

Love Your Slim Self helps you match your inside pictures to your outside image.

Remember the reading readiness papers kids got in kindergarten? They had to draw a line from one picture to whatever picture on the other side of the page was matching. The picture might have been a boy with a truck, a baby with a ball, or a dog with a bone.

The child might not know how to read the words: truck, ball or bone. It doesn't matter because the pictures tell the story and the child sees the connections and can match the pictures.

Sometimes there are trick pictures, a girl with a truck, a cat with a ball or a lion with a bone. The young learner who understands what the teacher wants doesn't fall for that trick and can make the connection to the correct image. The truck, the ball and the bone are the same regardless of the details.

As adults we match pictures all the time. It is how the brain works. When you go into a store with a clear idea of what you want or need you are using mental imagery. Perhaps you are looking for a black shirt. There isn't one in Store A. The picture in your mind is still vivid. You want a black shirt. If you keep the picture of a black shirt in your mind, you may go to another store, or you may go home without a shirt.

What if you decide to change the picture and a printed shirt or a blue shirt will do just as well?

AT THIS POINT, YOU CHANGE THE PICTURE INSIDE AND OUT.

You will see yourself in a printed shirt or a blue shirt and give up the desire to have a black shirt. The inner image is a powerful way to motivate change.

You can do the same thing with the picture of yourself. You can cling to the fat picture you have in your head, and stay fat outside, or you can **Love Your Slim Self** and change the picture inside first.

Changing the inner picture of yourself starts with an acceptance of who you are on the inside, no matter what outline the mirror shows you at this moment. By loving your self first, the picture of your slim self begins to become a real possibility and a reality.

Remember the black shirt you were shopping for? You may have looked at one, priced it, and even tried it on before you felt you were willing to change your desire for a black shirt and choose a different color. You were willing to change your mind and create a new possibility for the shirt.

With the outline of yourself in the mirror you may need to take some additional steps, see yourself as slim, believe that your inner self is slim and that you are on your way to catching up with the picture of yourself just the way you want to be.

You must have the right picture inside to create the desired effect outside. Athletes know the practice well. Golfers and tennis players learn to hold the inner picture to create the outer results. They have to see themselves winning the game. They build the confidence and a wall of belief that they can and do deserve to win. Their pictures are clear, detailed and specific and they match for success.

When it comes to slimness, for whatever reason, the inner picture is sometimes distorted, like a television view gone wrong or a film out of focus. The inner image must reflect the desired results of success.

Love Your Slim Self corrects the problem by correcting the image on the screen in your mind.

Take a breath...

"*To Love yourself right now, just as you are, is to give yourself heaven. Don't wait until you die. If you wait, your die now, If you love, you live now.*"

--Alan Cohen

CHAPTER 21
THEATER TICKETS
TO YOUR MIND

Here's proof you can visualize:

How many times have you browsed through a catalogue or read an ad and automatically pictured yourself wearing or using a product? Whether it's a garment, an appliance, or a tool, you wonder if you want or need it. It doesn't matter if you are a man or woman; your imagination creates a picture on your mind's movie screen.

While looking through a sports magazine, you might see yourself in a hunting jacket.

How would you look in that Halloween costume?

What adventures would you have in that safari outfit?

Are you looking for some comfortable pajamas?

How about a new warm winter coat?

With the changing seasons you might imagine a ride-on lawn mower or see yourself using that snow blower?

Each item you study brings its own set of reactions, and those reactions are exclusively yours.

Often you are not even aware of imagining your face or body appearing on the pages of the catalog or magazine, but you will react to the feelings and emotions the pictures initiate. That's why Madison Avenue has been so successful convincing us that sultriness and sexiness come in a shampoo bottle and that companionship and love come in a can of Coke.

Years ago cod liver oil needed no description to produce not only the memory of the awful taste, but the accompanying nauseous emotion as well. Automatic involvement!

When you glance through a clothing catalog you may see the same item pictured in a scratchy wool fabric or as a soft, smooth cashmere version.

Contrast the starched crisp shirt you might wear to work with the snuggly, flannel robe you're so happy to get into to enjoy a cozy evening at home.

Rejecting pictures also brings vivid images and, sometimes, clear feelings. Perhaps you want to plan a garden, so you decide not to order that thistle bush but choose the honeysuckle bush instead. Can you feel the thistles and predict the painful chore of planting? Can you smell the fragrant honeysuckle?

Which one have you chosen?

A skilled craftsman knows the weight of a tool by imagining how it will feel when he/she takes hold of the handle. In his mind's eye, he can predict how easily, or how badly, he can work with it. He may think, "This one will gouge the wood, while that one will carve smoothly."

The sea-lover can caress the hull of a boat or stand at the tiller and experience the spray of the ocean all in an imaginary scene. Even the land-lover can conjure the swell of the sea. If you have a tendency to get seasick, that feeling is one to move away from rather quickly.

Let's use the idea of someone who would rather not buy a boat because he or she is prone to getting seasick. For such a person, **"Not loving yourself,"** would mean being overcome by nausea.

"Just Being Yourself" would cause you to resolve not to become nauseous. **"Loving Your Slim Self"** would help you to think of dry land. As you begin to see **YOU**, your face, your body and your feelings as part of your visualization, you will begin to trust your inner wisdom. You will come to know the unconditional love only you can give to yourself.

One more aid can break through the strongest conditioning and immunity. If you've already gone through the "willing to be willing" exercise, and you still have conflicts, you might use the following exercise as a prescription to assist visualization.

Find a snapshot of yourself at your thinnest weight, and cut out your face, then paste the photo of your face in the center of a piece of blank paper or a piece of cardboard. Next, look through some magazines to find pictures you would want to be part of your future. This is you as your slim self and the pictures bring details to the possibilities of can happen in the future. If you can't find what you want in magazines, draw these scenes yourself. Cut them out and paste them around your face. Include pictures of where you might go on vacation, what kind of new car you would own, where would you love to live, what kind of house you want, etc.

Plan your future as your healthy vibrant, lovely slim self.

The next chapter is devoted to guiding you through new adventures in the aspects of feeling, seeing and knowing that are essential parts of **Love Your Slim Self**. Welcome to the theater of your mind. Here are your 3-D glasses. Settle back in your comfortable seat. You don't need popcorn.

"Your task is not to seek for LOVE, but merely to seek and find all the barriers within yourself that you have built against it."

--Rumi, thirteen century Sufi poet

CHAPTER 22
SEEING IS BELIEVING

What you see is what you get! No, no, not what you see in the mirror from the neck down, but what you see in your mind's eye. This process will unfold rather simply. Read this chapter, then sit comfortably in a chair, and close your eyes. Take five, deep belly breaths by inhaling through your nose, and slowly exhaling through your mouth. Feel yourself relax; then slowly count backwards from ten to one.

In your mind's eye, imagine yourself looking exactly as you want to look in the future. Too many people stop here. While this exercise is helpful, it's not specific enough. Now, add more details. You can never have too many details. You are without limitations.

For example, you can start like this:

"I see me as slim, attractive and buoyant. I'm walking on a beach wearing a light jacket. The wind is blowing and I can see beach umbrellas swaying. The temperature is balmy and delightful. The sun begins to warm me and I remove my jacket. I feel great in my swimsuit and am delighted with the sense of freedom and ease with which I continue walking down the beach. In fact, I look amazing in the picture in my mind and feel comfortable in my own skin."

Do you think you have sketched enough details? Nonsense. You've just begun. You have been practicing the seeing skill, but haven't yet added the emotion-packed part that will bring the picture to life, but do you notice how feelings have crept in already? Emotions just can't help showing up. Any picture you imagine will trigger emotion.

Now, let's intensify the emotion. It's just like making your computer screen brighter or changing the contrast. We'll continue with easy seeing.

What's the skyline in your picture? You might imagine the Florida Keys or the coast of France. It's your picture and your mind. Can you imagine the horizon and add details to the background so that you completely recognize the scene?

Notice the clean, white sand, and continue adding to your scene.

Smell the salt in the air, and detect the sweet scent of your sunscreen lotion. Then see yourself walk over to a nearby refreshment stand, choose a hotdog, take two small bites and throw the rest away.

Now, add even more life to the picture: "I begin to explore my feelings. I notice I am not experiencing any deprivation. I took those two bites of the hot dog and realized six more bites would taste just the same. Anyway, all I wanted was just one bite."

Adding feelings to your picture is vital. Think of all the jokes about smell-a-vision, they're not as far out as they once seemed. You've added both fragrance and emotion to your visualization. Practice it daily. As the scene begins to take permanent shape, **YOU** will begin to take shape in a new way. Soon you'll walk and talk differently without even noticing the change in yourself.

One sad thing about people who have lost 50 or 100 pounds is they have not fallen in love with their slimmer selves. In their everyday actions, most especially in their walk, they show they still feel fat.

Try this quick, easy experiment.

No matter what your present size is, tell yourself you are enormous, grossly overweight, many sizes greater than you ever were. Walk across the room. Feel the heaviness? See how hard it is to move one foot ahead of the other? You are huge as you lumber along. Perhaps your body hurts.

Now, **Love Your Slim Self**. Tell yourself you are your ideal weight. You are slim, trim, fit, and healthy. Walk, glide, or dance across the room in your new, light body.

How did you feel in the first action-picture? How did you feel in the second?

No matter what your present size, if you practice these strategies, you will begin to feel the change. But wait! Practice them **EASILY, COMFORTABLY, and LIGHTLY**; otherwise, you're forcing yourself and are not **Loving Your Slim Self**. Forcing something takes trying, and trying too hard sets you up for failure. **Love Your Slim Self** sets you up for success.

Paste the pictures of inspiration here!

"Love is the great miracle cure. Loving ourselves works miracles in our lives."

--Louise L. Hay

CHAPTER 23

BELIEVING IS ACHIEVING, ACTIVATE YOUR "ACT AS IF"

Once you understand how to "**ACTASIF**" you already are slim, doing so becomes so easy it will become one word. It will become such a part of you that some day, you will wonder when "**ACTASIF**" ended and the real change began.

"**ACTASIF**" begins in the pretend compartment of your mind. When you conceive, believe, breathe and achieve the ability to **Love Your Slim Self,** you will be moving in the right direction.

At some point, **Love Your Slim Self,** clicks into place and becomes an Aha moment after Aha moment!

Compare yourself to a person who desperately needs a job who is down to his or her last five dollars. If that individual drags himself into a job interview looking or FEELING needy, the vibe from that attitude and appearance may turn off a prospective employer. You would not make a positive impression on any employer when you are feeling so needy.

In today's sophisticated world, John and Joan, job seekers, dress the part. Maybe Joan's last five dollars goes towards a bright scarf, or a fresh flower, and John goes towards a new tie. Already, with these purchases, John and Joan feel better. The air is charged with more positive ions, and the interviewer can't help feeling their positive vibes.

Their purchases represent a confidence in the faith they have in themselves. Their positive attitude will not guarantee the new job.

But, they'll feel G-R-E-A-T!

Many a self-made millionaire will testify to using these same tactics to reach his or her goal. **"ACTASIF"** you are already there.

One way to strengthen your **"ACTASIF"** is to research how slim people react around food.

Slim people detest feeling full. After slim people finish eating, they will not take one more bite, even when asked to.

Consider the idea of not liking the feeling of being too full. You do not have to do anything differently; just consider the thought. When you are ready, you may **Love Your Slim Self** into a new way of thinking.

To make an analogy, consider your mind like a computer. By changing the hard drive you can re-boot for more effective programming. Consider changing the pattern or mindset of your inner pictures and internal dialogue. Your ability to be aware of these new ideas will begin to support your efforts towards success.

Now that you are aware of **"ACTASIF"**, this story will make an interesting point.

> Frank talked constantly about his inability to stop eating. One day he started to feel somewhat full, and his plate was almost empty, but he just couldn't put down his fork and leave the rest. He kept shoveling in the food. He said he "wasn't slim yet' and that right now, he'd "rather not do anything about it." When he remembered to think about what slim people do, and to actually pretend that he was already slim, it was easier for him to stop eating. He even threw away some of the meal.

He was actually able to "**ACTASIF**" he was an actor on the stage of life.

And didn't Shakespeare make that the truth:

> **"All the world's a stage**
>
> **And all the men and women merely players**
>
> **They have their exits and their entrances**
>
> **And one man in his time plays many parts…."**

"**ACTASIF**" you have your name on the marquee as the star of the show. You are important and it is only you that can feel the love for yourself in order to play the new role of **Loving Your Slim Self.**

"To love oneself is the beginning of a life-long romance."

--Oscar Wilde

"Man often becomes what he believes himself to be. If I keep on saying to myself that I cannot do a certain thing, it is possible that I may end up really becoming incapable of doing it. On the contrary, if I have the belief that I can do it, I shall surely acquire the capacity to do it even if I may not have it at the beginning."

--Mahatma Gandhi

CHAPTER 24

WHALES

Now it's time to take stock. I predict you will be both surprised and pleased.

What's happened to you since you began reading this book? You were not asked to work, only to remain aware and to take notice. Take a few minutes to relax and ask yourself what changes have taken place in your relationship with food, in your relationship with yourself?

People recovering from certain illnesses rejoice at the smallest perceptible movement of a toe. Gradually, if they are lucky, with more training and practice, they begin to make further progress. Changes in you may be subtle but if you can identify them, you will reinforce the promise of further change.

No matter how infinitesimal you perceive changes to be, they still are life-changes and you can congratulate yourself wholeheartedly. Before you began to adopt the **Love Your Slim Self** principles, you were conditioned to consider some changes so insignificant that you ignored them. With your new awareness, however, you will be able to spot small, but significant changes.

Here's a visual experience that might help you understand the significance of looking for changes that will reinforce your success.

Have you ever been on a whale-watching cruise? Of course, you want to see the whales, but first, the guide must prepare you for the adventure. At the start of the cruise, you will hear about the habits of whales, where they are headed, and why you are going to a good place to see them. Sometimes, you may hear stories of previous sightings and even may see educational videos about whales, learn their history, and witness their grace and beauty.

Then, as you approach the site, your guide will bring the group together and exclaim enthusiastically, "We're nearing the site, so everyone look for a flock of birds!"

BIRDS? What? How far from whales can you get? Up in the air? A different species altogether? Why would you look for something so foreign from your goal of watching whales?

The birds will give you the clue that something is moving under the water. Soon, you will see the spout that signifies the creature itself. Finally, the surfacing of the whale brings the excitement that accompanies the sighting.

If you are not paying attention to the birds or to the spout, you will miss seeing the whale. You, your brain, and your vision just aren't fast enough to simply "look" for the whale. First, you must know what to look for. If you miss the signs, you will miss the whale.

Inexperienced watchers rarely see these signs until the guide points them out. Because they weren't aware of the meaning of what to watch for, they missed the signs, and the opportunity to see the whales.

Remember, you looked for birds, then saw a spout, and finally, you saw the whale. You came prepared with layers of clothing. You did not spot every whale or every sign, but you witnessed enough so that no matter how many whales you see in the future, whether at an aquarium, an amusement or a water park, you will remember the excitement and adventure of whale watching on the ocean.

With **Love Your Slim Self**, you also have been preparing for an adventure. Right now, you're in the "watching area."

But once you start paying strict attention, once you start to spot the correct signs, you will see the personal and individual changes only you can identify.

Some changes take place with little conscious effort. These are the behavioral changes that result from feeling changes and that's why you hardly notice them. For each change you do notice, give yourself a gold star, or two or three. You're in charge of the box of gold stars.

Do whatever it takes to acknowledge movement toward your goal to **Love Your Slim Self**. Once you have an intrinsic sense of accomplishment, you will find "gold stars" everywhere!

Have you noticed the small signs? At any time since you started this book, have you noticed you have:

Postponed eating something you thought you would like?

Closed the refrigerator door when you were just looking without removing anything?

Left the room when the desire for food arose?

Left the house?

Looked in the mirror and gave yourself a positive pat?

Became aware that for a moment you thought you were hungry, but you let the moment pass?

Ate less sugar during the day?

Parked your car further away than usual?

Drank water instead of diet soda?

Walked up the stairs instead of taking the elevator?

Took a glass of water to see if that twinge was really hunger or thirst?

Made your own observations?

Congratulated yourself on small changes?

You and your body, especially with your new awareness, have information that far surpasses any knowledge you have gained from this book. Once the mind has adopted a new idea, it will not revert to a thought that no longer works.

The attitude that results if you **Love Your Slim Self** will begin to trigger the actions and behaviors that validate your changes, not only in the here and now, but also for your future success.

Tom had an aversion to the taste of coffee. In fact, it would make him sick, but he loved the aroma. It didn't take him long to realize that he could **simply** (notice simply) inhale the scent of his favorite brew.

Take the case of a "popcorn princess." Tina loved the smell of movie popcorn, but she did not enjoy the taste. Now, she simply feasts on the aroma and enjoys the movie.

If the sizzle sells the steak, consider how to feel full from the sizzle.

It's all in your mind anyway!

CHAPTER 25

HOLD THAT LINE

HOLD THAT LINE, or **how to be your own cheering section.**

Have you ever noticed that when a football team is in danger of defeat, the cheer becomes "Hold that line, hold that line!" Even though the team may not get a touch down or progress at all, the cheerleaders and the fans applaud holding the line as if it were a victory!

What about when you "hold that line" in the face of great odds? When you maintain your weight? Nobody applauds and the truth is that you don't even applaud yourself.

Why not? No weight gain is a victory of sorts, and it is a truth that maintenance is the first step toward slimness.

At some moment of truth, people who maintain their weight will decide that if they did not gain weight, they still would be able to buy clothes. They stand with the rising determination to hold that line. Logically, the first step to losing weight is to maintain, to stop gaining. Once you **Love Your Slim Self** into a relaxed attitude about maintenance, you're on your way to your goal.

"Not to fall backwards is a way to advance, for man must first walk before he can dance." – Anonymous

"One of the bests guides to how to be self-loving is to give ourselves the love we are often dreaming about receiving from others. There was a time when I felt lousy about my over-forty body, saw myself as too fat, too this or too that. Yet I fantasized about finding a lover who would give me the gift of being loved as I am. It is silly, isn't it, that I would dream of someone else offering to me the acceptance and affirmation I was withholding from myself. This was a moment when the maxim "You can never love anybody if you are unable to love yourself" made clear sense. And I add, "Do not expect to receive the love from someone else you do not give yourself"

--bell hooks

CHAPTER 26
AS I MOVE AND BREATHE

The only exercise you must regularly do is **BREATHE**.

That's right...just breathe...in and out!

For many of us who are half a century or older, the first encounter with breathing occurred in the delivery room where you were surrounded by bright lights, noise and confusion. Today infants are ushered into the world with soft lighting, a calm environment, quiet voices and a nurturing birthing atmosphere. When entering the world, the baby finds the breath, begins to breathe with ease and comfort and settles in to begin the bonding process with mom.

If you have the opportunity to be around a newborn, quietly observe their breathing. Notice that when the baby is calm and resting, that the breath is full, easy and starts with the belly rising.

Let's review the instructions on how to breathe?

> Stop for a few seconds and pay attention to the air that comes in at the bottom of your nose. Now take a deep breath by filling your belly first and then allow the air to fill the rest of your chest. As you begin to exhale, allow the air to leave from the top of your lungs first and then to compress the rest of the air until your belly is empty again. As you exhale, imagine all the tightness and stress leaving your body.

The benefits that accompany breathing in this way will support many areas of your life. Take a deep full breath while you are waiting in traffic, at a red light or standing in line. Breathe consciously when someone asks you a question and you need more time to respond. Do it when you are feeling anxious, or sad or even frightened. Breathing can make the difference between reacting to something with upset and frustration or choosing to respond to something with thought and purpose.

NOW BREATHE... In and out

If that is all you can do consciously, then you are well on your way to changing your life. Remember to breathe, in and out, even saying those words to yourself.

"I am breathing in, and I am breathing out."

By being aware of your breathing throughout the day, you will have another strategy to assist in your desire to **Love Your Slim Self.** When you breathe with intention, you become mindful and present to what is happening in your body and in your environment. You are able to easily reduce stress, recharge your brain and your thinking and shift your emotional reactions to conscious purpose rather than old habits.

The next exercise is simple, natural movement. Take a breath, and reflect on how many times you **MOVE** during the day, how you move, where you move, what moves you make.

When you begin the process of **Loving Your Slim Self**, movement becomes an activity you begin to cherish and appreciate. Remember, awareness is the first step toward change, and once you realize the importance of small changes, you will begin to move your body with grace.

When you shop in the grocery store, go for a stroll, climb the stairs, go bowling with the kids, swim in a pool, do the laundry or vacuum the rugs, you are moving. Recognize movement as an essential part of caring for yourself, so that movement will become fun and entertaining.

Have you ever watched a broadcast of an exercise class? Did you notice the leader's motivating words? These leaders know how to make movement comfortable and easy.

Richard Simmons is a blast from the past and has been around for the past 30 years helping people learn to have fun while moving.

In an open letter to his fans he says:

"I want you to keep dancing with me. I want you to keep nourishing your body with the right foods and in the right-size portions. I want you to keep loving yourself. And I want you to always know that you're worthy of being healthy, for the rest of your life."

If you have been advised against vigorous exercise because of medical reasons, it's all the more reason to celebrate the moves you do make. Walking around the house or climbing a few stairs, moving your arms, hands and feet periodically throughout the day is a beginning for movement. As you find ingenious ways to move comfortably within the framework of your medical condition you will discover that limitations can become challenges. If you look around your world, just as whale watchers search for the birds, you will notice many people moving to the best of their ability.

Just do more moving yourself!

Beverly found a new way of moving when her son gave her a pair of sunglasses with a CD player built into the frame. The music was literally "ringing in her ears" and she had no choice but to move and dance. The music was so inspiring and fun, that her head was filled with the motivation she needed to move her body. And dance she did, as she made the beds, cleaned the kitchen, straightened the living room and cooked dinner. At 77 years young, she found a new way of loving herself while she had a blast moving through her day.

Share your innovative and creative ways of moving with people you care about. Make a list for yourself so you will always have ideas available. Playing the computer (doesn't that sound like more fun than just typing?) and even pencil-pushing as opposed to push-ups, both count. That's easy, simple, comfortable movement. When you acknowledge the little movements, it is "**Time to give yourself more gold stars.**"

TAKE NOTE: Have you noticed the absence of chapters about exercise, food plans, and calories? Here in the **Love Your Slim Self** world, your change happens as a result of a new mindset.

Calories do count, but they are to be put into perspective. You can calculate calories; you can recognize them but for heaven's sake, don't labor over them. Very few of you are virgin dieters. Virgin dieters pour over calorie lists or obsess over rigid food lists. While they may lose weight by following "the rules," most of the time they will regain more weight than they lost.

As an experienced weight-loser, you know every calorie in that same book. You may have blocked them out but now, in your new-relaxed mode of **Loving Your Slim Self** that knowledge will work for you. The change in your behavior will work in concert with your ability to awaken your loving self.

You have begun to communicate with your body and to trust your inner self to the point where you know that all the shifting and sifting can be done automatically in that built-in computer of your mind. Agonizing about calories only limits that process.

It's the same way with compulsive, grit your teeth and force yourself exercise. Movement is fun! Moving is stretching luxuriously; moving is getting out of bed in the morning; moving is running to meet your lover; moving is dancing to commercials, moving is bending down to pick up your grandchild, and above all, moving is changing, which is what **Love Your Slim Self** is all about.

"Optimism is the faith that leads to achievement. Nothing can be done without hope and confidence."
--Helen Keller

"There are two basic motivating forces: fear and love. When we are afraid, we pull back from life. When we are in love, we open to all that life has to offer with passion, excitement, and acceptance. We need to learn to love ourselves firs, in all our glory and our imperfections. If we cannot love ourselves, we cannot fully open to our ability to love others or our potential to create. Evolution and all hopes for a better world rest in the fearlessness and open-hearted vision of people who embrace life."

--John Lennon

___

CHAPTER 27
COMMENCEMENT ROSE

Old thinking is a rose with thorns. Negative thinking is a plastic rose. New thinking is **Love Your Slim Self**, a fresh rose in all its fragrance, a thorn-less beauty, shaped by your desire for change.

EASY and **COMFORTABLE** thinking will bring you your Commencement Rose, the **Love Your Slim Self** rose. See yourself accepting it as you graduate into your new way of life.

Originally, the word "diet" meant a way of life. It was a perfectly neutral word before it took on emotionally packed connotations. Diet is a word that triggers all kinds of fears below the surface. We think deprivation, starvation, struggle, pain and suffering. The word **DIET** became distorted, and for decades, people have been put off because of the first three letters "DIE."

ENOUGH! Love Your Slim Self is about living your life with ease and comfort and with fun and delight. You will come to understand, and rely on your inner knowing. In your mind, in your heart and in your body, you absolutely know what is right for your health and well-being. Trusting yourself is just another step in your journey to accepting that, indeed, you do **Love Your Slim Self,** unconditionally!

Learn to **Love Your Slim Self** when you are in the company of well-intentioned friends and family who may think they are only helping you when they say:

What diet are you on NOW?

Is that on your diet?

I thought you were trying to lose weight!

Won't your mother be pleased?

Be careful. George, or Nancy, or your cousin Maude will be jealous.

You look twenty years younger.

How did you ever let yourself go like that?

You are stronger now than you were before. You know that no one can rock your world without your permission. You are in charge of how you feel and of how you respond.

Breathe, reframe your attitude, and simply acknowledge such comments with grace and say, "Thank you for noticing," or "Thank you for your support." Then walk away!

The good news is that for every hurt there is a healing. When you take responsibility for maintaining "right thought," "right speech," and "right action," everyone wins!

The secret is to leave the fragile scab in place. Recognize that healing is taking place and no bump caused by insensitive people can hurt the new you.

It's okay, in fact, it's vital to recognize people saying and making hurtful comments. Good intentions have nothing to do with it.

It doesn't matter if someone hurts you, either intentionally or not. If the bruise is there, it still hurts. When you **Love Your Slim Self**, you gather information that gives you a choice. You accept the inevitable, that you must eat less and move more, but you examine every way you do it, **EASILY** and **COMFORTABLY**.

When you **Love Your Slim Self**, you will notice ideas you never thought of before, especially when you re-read old material.

When you **Love Your Slim Self**, you will find books, resources and relationships that help you discover softer ways of dealing with yourself. You will find yourself giving yourself the same consideration you want from others.

NOW is the time.

NOW is the time to keep the tools and skills in your heart. **Breathe, S.O.S.**, and **ACTASIF** to allow yourself to feel good.

Feeling good doesn't depend on being rich, getting a new car, earning a degree or losing weight. A person who feels good about him/herself, and who isn't always waiting for something to happen first, **EASILY, COMFORTABLY,** and continuously lives joyously.

You are not looking to make your life perfect, only better. You will begin to make better choices that will lead to your joy: a slimmer you.

Avoid "gritting your teeth" for anything. Choose to smile instead of grimacing.

There is no magic, and if you are looking for the "It"...

...It's **YOU**.

Love Your Slim Self

Resources

Some of my favorite References, Resources and Amazing People

The Relaxation Response by Dr. Herbert Benson

The Miracle of the Breath, by Andy Caponigro

Full Catastrophe Living: Using the Wisdom of Your Body and Mind to Face Stress, Pain and illness, by Jon Kabat-Zinn

Jumping on Water by Ted Karam

Lighten Up, by Loretta LaRoche

The Tapping Solution by Nick Ortner

Savor: Mindful Eating, Mindful Life by Thich Nhat Hanh

www.Heartmath.com

www.mindfulschools.org

www.theamazingdogtrainingman.com

www.heartsongyoga.com

www.aliassolutions.com

www.thetappingsolution.com

Some of the people who helped and said: "You can do this"

A BIG GLORIOUS THANKS!

Beverly Klegraefe, Tim and Liz Frangioso, Eric and Rachael Letendre, Kristin Rotas, David Axelrad, Rachael Jacobson, Joyce Singer, Sherry Branch, Ellen Mills-Audette and Donna Hobart.

www.ingramcontent.com/pod-product-compliance
Lightning Source LLC
Chambersburg PA
CBHW071138280326
41935CB00010B/1283

* 9 7 8 0 9 8 4 4 4 5 0 0 4 *